LEONARD MCCRARY

The Parent Commandments

10 Principles for Raising Strong, Resilient Children

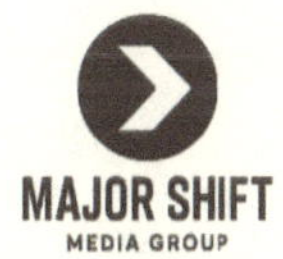

First published by Major Shift Media Group 2026

Copyright © 2026 by Leonard McCrary

All rights reserved. No part of this publication may be reproduced, stored, or transmitted in any form or by any means, electronic, mechanical, photocopying, recording, scanning, or otherwise without written permission from the publisher. It is illegal to copy this book, post it to a website, or distribute it by any other means without permission.

First edition

ISBN (paperback): 979-8-9938556-0-8
ISBN (hardcover): 979-8-9938556-1-5

This book was professionally typeset on Reedsy.
Find out more at reedsy.com

Contents

Dedication

To my dearest friend,

Brittney Hammond — "Ham & Cheese."

Many years ago, you saw this book in me before I ever put pen to paper.

Your motivation, laughter, and unwavering belief became the spark that ignited *The Parent Commandments.*

Thank you for pushing me to write what my heart had only whispered.

This book exists because you reminded me it was already inside me.

1

Thou Shalt Not Do Unto Them Kids, Just Because Thou Parents Did It Unto You

Call It What It Is

Breaking a generational curse means consciously choosing to disrupt the harmful patterns passed down through families, cycles like addiction, abuse, poverty, or toxic communication. It's more than what happened to us, it's also about what we choose to continue or heal. Breaking the cycle requires honesty, awareness, effort, and support. Often through therapy, community, or reflection. Listen, it's hard! But it's also rewarding. Because every choice to do better creates a new legacy. A legacy that's not shaped by struggle, but shaped by strength, consciousness, and love.

Let's keep it real for second. Some of the things our parents did to us? Wild. Yet here we are, grown and trying to parent in a completely different world. Still hearing our parents' voices flying out of our mouths like spiritual possession. "Because I said so." "Go to bed before I give you something to cry about." "You think I'm one of your little friends?" Truthfully, just because something was done to us, doesn't mean it should be repeated through us.

Growing up in my house, asking questions wasn't always allowed. My father's word was loud and it was law. He would often say, "Speak your mind!" but I learned quickly that it only seem to apply if my thoughts and ideas didn't challenge him. I thought freedom of speech existed, until I tried it. That contradiction planted seeds I'm still uncovering today. To cope with it, I journaled, I wrote songs, and I held my tongue.

So what does that look like now? At bedtime, you're triggered by your kid stalling, but it's not really about the bedtime. It's about feeling like you've lost control. During conflict, you say "Don't talk back," but what you really mean is "Don't make me feel unheard." When they show emotion, you call them dramatic or sensitive, but deep down, it stings because you weren't allowed the same grace and to feel the same emotions.

What I've Seen

Have your parents ever punished you as a kid and you later realize... they were just tired? My parents had trauma. They had pressure. They had bills, a lot of bills! They didn't have time to think about gentle parenting. Besides, my father was everything but gentle. And now I stand in front of my own children trying to find the balance of being firm and being gentle. Trying to be better, but sometimes, I feel that same heat rising in me. The hand doesn't raise, but the twitch? The pulsating in my temple? It's there. And now, I get it.

That's when I started asking myself. Am I doing this because it's right, or because it's familiar?

I remember getting yelled at for "backtalk" just for asking "Why?" I got scolded for smacking my teeth or blowing my breath when I was frustrated. Now my daughter asks why I yell so loud. I start to answer, and she cuts me off, "You sound like Grandpa when he's mad at you." And just like that, I realized, I had become the voice I used to fear. The voice I hated hearing.

Growing up in the '90s, basketball was everything to me and my friends. I could watch it all day and play it all day. It didn't matter if it were a video game, real life, or on the television. I truly lived at the court. But whenever I wanted to go play, I had to ask permission every single time. And the "no's" came often, without explanation, without reason. So I promised myself, when I have kids, I'll explain my decisions. Not because I owe it, but because I want them to understand, even if they don't always agree.

Sometimes, I don't even remember the punishment. I only remember being confined to my room and insulated in the deafening silence. The energy. The shame. My parents didn't have words like "emotional safety" or "regulation." But they gave what they had, often a short fuse wrapped in love. Occasionally I find myself passing that same fuse... unless I'm able to catch it. I learned to breathe. Pause. And say, "Give me a second." That's my code for, "I'm trying not to repeat what was passed down to me."

There was a day I heard my son pretend to be "the dad" while playing with his sisters. I was honored to see him imitating me, I mean I was his hero after all. That's when I heard him mimicking my angry voice, my posture, and my tone. In real time I was watching the behavior that I had modeled. That day shook me and made me feel awful. It was a gut check. I learned that kids not only repeat what you say, they also become what they see and what you embody.

However, I'm learning. And now when I mess up, I circle back. I apologize. I own it. I say things like, "You didn't deserve that tone," or "My bad, I was overwhelmed and I'm sorry." Not to make myself feel better, but to keep it all the way real with them and to show them that leadership includes humility. And that love doesn't excuse harm.

The Culture

Most of us may not have realized this, but we were raised on survival parenting. Yes our parents loved us deeply, but they were under pressure. They didn't have parenting podcasts, therapy apps, or emotional tool-kits. What they had was trauma passed down to them from generations unknown to us. So what we experienced as "discipline" was often control. Obedience was mistaken for respect, and emotional connection got lost in the shuffle.

Now? We're the first generation trying to do it differently. We are raising emotionally aware children while healing our own childhood wounds. We're parenting our children and re-parenting ourselves. It's exhausting but necessary. It's humbling and it's also courageous. We're the turning point. This change feels special, intentional, and generational.

Language That Builds Connection

Authority doesn't have to and shouldn't silence curiosity. You can say, "Here's why I'm saying no", instead of, "Because I said so." You can say, "It's okay to cry", instead of, "Stop crying." You can say, "You seem upset, do you want space or want to talk?", instead of, "Fix your face."

Changing the language, changes the experience. And when you change the experience, you change the legacy. This type connection isn't built overnight. You have to be prepared to put in the work, even when it's uncomfortable. Even when you're angry and your patience is at an all time low. I've learned to take this one conversation at a time.

Try this exercise: Say This, Not That

Say this: 'Surviving something doesn't mean I have to repeat it.'

Not That: 'My parents did it to me!'

Say this: 'I'm still unlearning some things.'

Not That: 'I turned out fine!'

Say this: 'Strength doesn't require suffering.'

Not That: 'Children today are too soft!'

The Mirror Moment

This is absolutely *not* about throwing away everything our parents did. It's about keeping the good, and breaking the harm. They gave what they had, what they could. Now we get to choose what continues through us, and what ends with us.

The shift is in the pause, gathering your composure, and taking a breath. The "Give me a second." The apology. The effort. The awareness. This is what breaking a cycle looks and feels like. Nothing overly dramatic, instead it's intentional.

Understand that you are the ancestor now. You are the blueprint maker. The cycle shifter. The one who said, "It ends here." This work is not only important, it's also pioneering and the start of a new legacy for generations to come.

Reflection + Challenge

This week, challenge yourself. Pause before you react. Catch the script. Break it. Rewrite it.

Questions to Reflect On:

1. What's something I swore I'd never do that I find myself repeating?
2. What behavior from my child triggers a strong reaction in me, and why?
3. What would the younger me have needed in that moment?
4. How can I show up differently this week?

Challenge:

Breathe. Pause. Choose differently. Say it out loud: "It ends with me."

The Amen

Breaking the cycle doesn't make you disloyal to your parents nor does it mean you're abandoning your past. It simply means you're committed to your future. It doesn't erase your parents' sacrifices, it just means you believe some things can and should be done differently. This is why I chose reflection over reaction. I choose healing over habit. I choose intention over tradition.

And that, right there, is the start of generational change. May your parenting be rooted in wholeness, and not wounds. Amen.

2

Thou Shalt Say No to Thy Kids, Just Because Thou Can

Call It What It Is

Let's keep it "one hundred," most of us tell our children 'yes' only because we heard 'no' so many times growing up. We don't want our children to feel the same disappointments we felt so we tend to bend the knee and oblige to their wants and demands. It doesn't help that we live in a world that whispers 'yes' into our kids' ears all day long. Ads, apps, influencers, and peers all saying, "You should have more, be more, buy more." And when we say 'no' as parents, it feels like we're snatching the air out of the room.

Truthfully, you are allowed to say no, with love, with peace, and with no explanation. In fact, it might be one of the most important parenting tools you have. Now I know this may sound contradicting from what I said earlier about giving my children an explanation when I say no. But lets not get it twisted, I'm in charge. I give them an explanation because I want them to have an understanding. However, I don't owe anything. If I choose to only say no and walk away like the toughest guy in an old western movie, then so be it.

Saying no doesn't make you mean. It makes you mindful. Our job isn't to shield our kids from every disappointment, it's to teach them how to sit with it. To feel it. To move through it without collapsing. Whenever we constantly say yes to avoid their frustration, we rob them of the muscle they'll need later in life, the ability to hear "no" and still know they're loved, safe, and whole. That's a skill. And like any skill, it's built through practice, even if that practice starts in the cereal aisle.

"No" teaches boundaries. "No" teaches discernment. "No" teaches the difference between needs and wants. And when it's delivered with steadiness and love, instead of shame or power, it becomes a gift. Not just for your child, but for the future version of them who will have to navigate jobs, relationships, deadlines, rejections, and life itself. Saying no isn't withholding love at all. It's actually shaping wisdom.

So the next time you feel guilty for saying no, remember this. You're not taking something away. You're giving something deeper. You're giving them the ability to wait and the ability to trust. To accept limits without losing themselves. And in a world that constantly screams more, now, yes, your steady "no" might just be the most loving thing they hear all day.

What I've Seen

One day my son asked for a $300 vintage video game on a random Tuesday. No birthday. No honor roll. Just vibes. I said, "No." He said,"'But you have money." I replied, "I also have sense. And just because you got it, doesn't mean 'you got it!"

The blank look. The look of disappointment. The silent cold stare spoke loudly. But it didn't move me one bit.

Another time, my three year old daughter cried because I said no to ice cream at 9 AM. Surprisingly, I stayed calm, but inside I was spiraling, 'Should I just say yes? Am I too strict?'

On a different occasion I got a call from the teacher that my nine year old daughter was misbehaving in school. As punishment I didn't allow her to participate with her cheer team the same evening. Cue meltdown. Full protest. Pacing and breathing like I'd committed a federal offense.

Then there was my daughter's senior prom, a milestone moment I knew she'd remember for the rest of her life. I wanted it to be magical, a night she could look back on with joy. But when she told me she wanted to ride all over town with a young man I'd only met once over Face time, my fatherly instincts kicked in. All I could think about were the risks. Teenage driving, late-night distractions along with the other unknowns I couldn't control. As much as I wanted her to feel free, I knew my job wasn't to make her happy in that moment, it was to keep her safe. I knew saying no might make me the villain that night, but my parenting isn't about popularity or being liked. Sometimes the hardest part is protecting them from their own blind spots. So I told her no. Eventually, we worked out a compromise, the driving would be shared between the young man's mother and myself. It wasn't perfect, but it was safe, and she still got her moment.

That's when I remembered. Giving *in* doesn't prevent disappointment. It just delays it, and teaches my children that love means never hearing 'no.' Totally unrealistic.

I used to think saying no would damage the relationship, like love was this fragile thing that could shatter if I didn't bend to every request. But what I'm learning, over and over, is that the real damage comes when I abandon my boundaries to avoid their feelings. Their disappointment is not a sign I failed as a parent. It's just a sign they're simply human. It's a signal that they're having a hard time accepting limits and my job is to help guide them through that, not erase the limit itself.

There's a moment after every meltdown, after the slammed door, the teary protest, the dramatic silence, when the energy settles. In that stillness, connection is possible again. That's when we talk. That's when I say, "I know you're hurt. I know you're disappointed. But I made that decision because I love you enough to say no." I've found that those quiet recovery moments are just as powerful as the boundary itself. It's not the no that hurts them, it's when the no comes with coldness, chaos, and inconsistency. But when it comes with compassion, they learn resilience and relationship.

I replay the scenes in my head often. The ones where I gave in, and the ones where I stood firm. It's not the tears or the tantrums that haunt me, it's the times I said yes when everything in me knew I should've said no. Not because the request was outrageous, but because my yes was rooted in fear. Fear of being too harsh. Fear of being "like" my parents. Fear of them not liking me. That's when I have to remind myself, parenting isn't about being liked in the moment, it's about being trusted over time. And trust is something I truly cherish.

So I'm writing a new story, one where love is firm and kind. One where "no" isn't the end of connection, but the beginning of a deeper kind of trust. My children won't always get what they want, but they'll always know they are safe, seen, and loved. And if I have to be the "bad guy" for a day so they can be a better person for a lifetime, I'll take that trade every time.

Why It's Hard to Say No

Many of us grew up with too many no's and not enough

explanation. Or we grew up with parents who said yes to everything and we saw them burn out.

Now we alternate between guilt and exhaustion. We want to give them what we didn't have. We must know it's not cruel to have boundaries, it actually shows you care. Saying yes out of guilt may make them happy in the moment, but it also makes them entitled.

Boundaries don't and shouldn't block connection, they should protect it. When our children know we'll say no when needed, they feel safer, and not stifled. It shows them that love doesn't mean overextending yourself. It means being available with clarity, even when it's uncomfortable. Because if love always says yes, it stops being love and starts becoming performance.

Honestly, sometimes the yes isn't for them, it's for us. We say yes because we're tired. We say yes because we're afraid of the meltdown. We say yes because we don't want to feel like the "mean" parent. But parenting rooted in guilt leads to resentment. It builds a relationship where kids feel empowered, and parents feel depleted. It's like losing balance, and discovering self-abandonment.

We have to learn to sit with our children's disappointment without rescuing them from it. We have to let them be upset sometimes. Let them cry. Let them stomp away. Because those moments won't break the bond, if anything, they'll strengthen it. Children don't need perfection, they need consistency. They need to know you'll love them enough to hold the line.

So when you say no, do it with compassion. Do it with eye contact. Do it with a calm voice and a steady heart. Stand on it! Remind yourself, this boundary is love in action. Not the soft, sugar-coated kind. The kind that says, "I care enough to disappoint you today so you can be prepared for life tomorrow."

This type of parenting is tough but it's authentic. That's the kind that lasts.

How This Shows Up

It starts small. You say yes to something you didn't want to, and then find yourself "crashing out" later, not because your child did anything wrong, but because deep down, you're resentful. Resentful that your needs were ignored, but mostly because *you* ignored them. Other times, you feel guilty for saying no to something minor, like snacks before dinner or another episode before bed, so you over correct later. Now you're handing out extra screen time, buying toys, or easing up on a rule just to balance the emotional scales. But guilt is a poor guide for consistency.

Then there's the explaining. You say no, but instead of holding the line, you start over-explaining. You talk yourself into a corner while they chip away with more questions, more push back, more "please." Before you know it, you're worn down and saying yes to something you didn't mean to agree to in the first place. Or maybe you skip all that and go straight to bribing. "If you clean up, I'll give you a treat," or "Just do this one thing and I'll let you stay up late." It feels easier in the moment, but over time, it teaches them that limits are negotiable and love always comes with a payoff. Now you've gone from discipline to survival mode. And that can be terribly exhausting.

You say yes, then resent them for taking too much. You feel guilty saying no to small things, so you over correct later. You say 'no,' then explain yourself into a corner until they wear you down. You start bribing instead of setting boundaries.

Try this exercise: Say This, Not That

Say this: 'I'm saying no, and I know you're disappointed. That's okay.'

Not That: 'Because I said so.'

Say this: 'Asked and answered. Let's move on.'

Not That: 'Stop asking!'

Say this: 'No, not today.'

Not That: 'Maybe later' (knowing it's a no).

The Mirror Moment

Discipline starts with consistency. That consistency is included in your no. You don't need to yell. You don't need to negotiate. As my father would say, "You just need to say what you mean and mean what you say."

Boundaries are a love language. And 'no' is one of the most sacred ways you teach your child respect, patience, and self-control.

Don't get it misconstrued, you're not being harsh, you're being clear. When your child knows that your 'no' is steady and firm, and not spiteful and frantic, they learn to trust you. Deeper than that, they learn to trust themselves in a world that won't always say yes. Every time you hold a boundary with love, you're building their emotional muscle, and your own. Don't mistake control with leadership. That's the shift.

Reflection + Challenge: It's Time To Do The Work

They won't remember every toy you didn't buy. But they will remember how you taught them to hear 'no' without losing themselves. Say no with love. Say no with confidence. Say no, because you can. They'll thank you later, even if they protest now.

1. When was the last time I said 'yes' just to avoid a meltdown?
2. What part of saying 'no' makes me uncomfortable? Guilt, fear, rejection?
3. What does a healthy boundary look like in my home?
4. What is one small thing I can say 'no' to this week? Calmly and clearly?

Challenge: Try saying 'no' once this week without apologizing or over explaining. Then reflect on how your child responded and how you felt afterward.

Top 5 Wildest Things My Kids Have Asked For

1. A mansion with a water slide attached to their bunk bed.
2. A baby sibling specifically from Beyoncé.
3. $1,000 in cash to start a slime business.
4. A pet tiger that sleeps in their bed.
5. To quit school and become a Roblox YouTuber full-time.

Moral of the Story: Kids don't dream small. And it's okay to say no with a straight face and a soft heart.

The Amen

Every "no" rooted in love is a "yes" to their growth. Stand firm, speak truth, and trust that boundaries build blessings. It's natural for your conscience to tap your shoulder and guilt to settle in your chest, especially when your child's face drops or tears follow. But think of your "no" as a small deposit into their character bank. With time, consistency, and love, those deposits add up, and the return on that investment will be a strong, grounded child who knows limits, respect, and resilience.

The balance may not show up overnight, but one day, the interest will be undeniable.

3

Thou Shalt Not Use Thy Kids as Leverage or as a Bargaining Tool

Call It What It Is

Parenting is not a game of poker and your child is not a chip. Their love is not a tool and their needs are not leverage. But let's "keep it a buck", sometimes without even noticing, we turn parenting into negotiation, manipulation, or control.

Let's all say it together: Our kids are not pawns, not prizes, not proof, not props. They are not bargaining chips in a custody battle. They are not our emotional support pet when we're beefing with our partner. They are not leverage in an argument, or weapons in a war they didn't sign up for.

Unfortunately, you'd be surprised how many parents, good ones, loving ones, still use their kids to control, punish, or validate. It's not always loud. Sometimes it's subtle. "Tell your daddy I said..." "If you don't act right, I'm calling your mama." "Oh, you wanna stay with your other parent now? Fine. Go ahead."

What's meant to sting the other adult, often hits the child first.

Parenting is not a performance, it's a responsibility. Our children deserve to be raised in the safety of our maturity, not the mess of our unresolved emotions. They are not here to pick sides, carry messages, or prove loyalty. They are here to grow, to be loved, and to witness what love looks like when it's whole. So let's be the adults, even if we weren't perfectly parented, because they're watching, and we are their blueprint.

What I've Seen

I remember being in a mall and hearing a mom say to her child who appeared to be no more than six years old, "If you don't hug me, I'm not taking you to the park." And I froze, I recognized that language. I had said things like that. I had withheld things. I had flipped privileges into punishments and made affection conditional.

Another time, I told my daughter, "I guess I just do everything for this family and no one appreciates it." She looked crushed. She wasn't being ungrateful, she was being an eight year old. In that split second, I saw it clearly, I wasn't parenting, I was guilt-tripping. That's leverage disguised as language. And that's not the type of love I want to project.

Let me "tell on myself" for a second. Years ago, I was frustrated. My co-parent put me on child support and it absolutely crushed me. I was hurt. I was embarrassed. I felt like it was an indictment on my fatherhood. I felt like she was saying I wasn't showing up. And in that pain mixed with anger, I started parenting from a place of ego instead of love. I wanted to prove something, to her, to the system, even to myself. But the truth is, my children didn't need a performance, they just needed me to be present. They needed peace. And I had to learn that being a father isn't about control, money, or pride, it's about consistency, compassion, and showing up even when it's hard. Especially when it's hard.

So one day, when my kids asked me to take them to Disney World, it broke something deep inside me, because I knew I couldn't give them the magic they were asking for. My pockets were just as sad as I was. I whispered softly, "Not right now." My daughter looked up and asked, "Why?" And without thinking, I snapped, "Ask your mom!" The words hit the air before I could catch them. And in the silence that followed, I realized I had let my pain speak louder than my parenting.

Responding to my daughter from a place of bitterness, I saw the way her and her brother's faces dropped. I saw how they quietly carried that weight over the years, thinking it was theirs to hold. I wish I had truly realized, in that moment, what I was doing and the impact it would have. That's when I understood, even when I'm right, I can still be wrong. Unfortunately, this was only the beginning of a pattern that would repeat itself for years. And that's the hardest part, not fully understanding that I was planting seeds I never meant to grow.

I remember one time my friend told me about his six year old son coming home in tears. Why? Because he asked his mom if he could stay at Dad's house an extra night and his mom looked him dead in the eye and said, "I guess you love him more than me, huh?"

SIX. YEARS. OLD.

That child spent the rest of the week trying to "make it up" to his mom. Bringing her snacks. Laughing extra hard at her jokes. All because his little heart believed he'd done something wrong by having love.

When you use your kids to punish your co-parent, you don't hurt the other adult, you teach the child that love can be dangerous. That loyalty is a trap. That their heart is a battlefield where grown-ups come to settle scores. You blur the lines between safety and survival, and suddenly, the people they trust most become the ones they fear disappointing. The damage doesn't show up right away, but it echoes for years. And by the time you see it, they've already learned to flinch at love.

Why It Happens

Hurt people try to hurt back. Breakups, especially with kids involved, are emotionally intense. When someone feels betrayed, abandoned, or disrespected, they might use the only "power" they feel they have left, access to the child, to strike back. It's not about the child. It's about the wound.

Losing a relationship can feel like losing control. And when the relationship is over but the parenting isn't, some people try to control something, schedules, visitation, communication, to feel like they still have a grip on what's falling apart.

Some parents use their kids as "proof", to show the world, or themselves, that they're the "better" parent. That the child chooses them, sides with them, loves them more. It's not always intentional, but it happens when identity gets wrapped up in the pain. If someone grew up watching manipulation or emotional blackmail in their own home, they might repeat those behaviors without even realizing it. It becomes the default script, "this is just how people act when love goes bad."

Sometimes, parents are still operating from their own unmet needs and inner child wounds. They don't have the emotional tools to separate their personal feelings from their parenting responsibilities.

But here's the tragic part. The child becomes collateral damage. They're forced to navigate adult emotions they didn't cause and can't fix. And that's a heavy burden to grow up with.

The weight doesn't just fall out of nowhere, it's passed down. Often unintentionally. Parents don't wake up and decide to wound their children. They repeat what they know. The dysfunction gets disguised as love, and the manipulation gets masked as protection.

We learned these behaviors from somewhere. We saw it in families that praised silence and obedience, not expression or autonomy. We internalized the idea that love must be earned, that affection is transactional, and that control equals care.

So we say things like: "If you keep acting like that, you won't get anything from me." "Go hug your grandma or you won't get dessert." "After everything I've done for you..."

But what we think is discipline becomes emotional currency, and our kids start to believe their worth is performance-based.

How This Shows Up

There was a time I thought I was just "teaching a lesson." When my child made a mistake, I'd withdraw, emotionally, physically, spiritually. I wouldn't say much, but the air between us would turn cold. Or I'd say too much, the kind of words laced with guilt instead of guidance. I'd compare them to their siblings, or to the version of them I thought they should've been. I'd remind them how disappointed I was, hoping it would sting just enough to change them. I thought I was parenting. But if I'm honest with myself, I was punishing, not with spankings or timeouts, but with emotional distance. With silence. With shame. And I only realized later that what I was really doing was parenting the way I had been parented.

I've been reflecting on that, deeply. Because when I strip away the noise, I don't want my kids to fear my disapproval more than they trust my love, like I did with my parents, especially with my dad. I don't want them to walk on eggshells just to avoid "messing up." That's not discipline. That's emotional manipulation. And that type of manipulation doesn't teach a lesson, it only leaves a scar.

These days I ask myself: Am I guiding or guilt-tripping? Am I modeling emotional control, or just reacting from my own childhood wounds? Because if discipline doesn't teach love, patience, and repair, it's just punishment dressed up in authority.

My kids don't need a perfect parent. But they do need a consistent one. One that's available. One who can say: "You were wrong. But you're still safe. You're still loved. And we're going to get through this together."

Try this exercise: Say This, Not That

Say this: "Let's calm down together. I'm not going anywhere."

Not That: "If you don't stop crying, I'm leaving you here."

Say this: "You never have to hug anyone to get something from me."

Not That: "You better give me a hug or I'm not buying that toy."

Say this: "We're all lucky to have each other, even when we're frustrated."

Not That: "Do you know how lucky you are to have me?" (during a disagreement)

The Mirror Moment

You don't need to weaponize your love to raise strong children. You need consistency, grace, boundaries, and unconditional presence. Don't parent for power, parent for relationship.

This was most of my childhood experience growing up with my father. Everything seemed to be about control. And if he felt like he didn't have control he would make sure you and everyone else knew who was head honcho.

I'll admit the intimidation factor from my dad and the idea of making him angry did indeed keep me in line. Ironically, once I became a father I wanted to take some of that same approach. I wanted my kids to fear upsetting or disappointing me in hopes it would keep them from making bad decisions. In hindsight, they didn't need to fear me at all. They just needed to know that I genuinely cared about them. They would come to know that through the relationships and trust that I had built with them.

Healthy parenting isn't about forcing gratitude. It's about modeling unconditional connection. The relationship between you and your children isn't a popular app, it shouldn't come with terms and conditions. Discipline teaches behavior. But love? Love teaches identity. And when they know they are loved without performance, they become free to grow.

When we start using our kids as emotional leverage, punishing them with silence, making them pick sides in adult battles, or dangling our love like a prize, we're not parenting, we're controlling. And control, masquerading as love is one of the most dangerous lessons a child can learn. It teaches them that affection must be earned, that conflict must be feared, and that love disappears when people disappoint you. Some of us, myself included, are still healing from those lessons ourselves. So let's break that cycle. Your child should never be the middleman in your unresolved pain, not with your partner, not with their other parent, and definitely not with you. They're not pawns in your power struggle. They're people, watching, learning, and quietly asking, "Will love still find me, even when I'm hard to love?" Your answer, with your words and your actions, is their blueprint for the world.

Reflection + Challenge

1. Have I ever used love or affection as a tool to get compliance?
2. Do I guilt my child into gratitude or affection?
3. When was the last time I gave love without condition, even when they were 'misbehaving'?

Challenge: Say "I love you" during a moment of tension. Give a hug when they least 'expect' it. Model the unconditional care you want them to believe in.

Reminder: What Kids Learn from Leverage

- Love can be taken away.
- My worth depends on how I act.
- Guilt is how I make things right.

And as adults, they may:

- Struggle with boundaries.
- Become people-pleasers.
- Mistake control for love.

Break that cycle now, while their hearts are still soft and open.

The Amen

Children are not chess pieces, they are souls entrusted to your care. Love them without conditions. Protect their peace like it's sacred. Let your love be steady, not strategic, and your intentions pure. Don't dangle affection or rewards as bargaining chips, and don't send the message that love is something they have to work for or prove they deserve. If the relationship between you and your partner has soured, do everything in your power to keep the children out of the crossfire. They weren't part of that bond, and they shouldn't bear the weight of a breakup they didn't cause. Your job isn't to pull them closer to you or further from the other parent, it's to keep them whole.

4

Thou Shalt Not Swim in Guilt for Putting Thyself First Occasionally

Call It What It Is

You can't pour from an empty cup, but parents are out here scraping the bottom, handing out drops like it's noble. Self-care isn't selfish, and rest isn't a reward, it's a requirement. You are a human, not a martyr. And your kids don't need a burnt-out version of you with a smile painted on. They need a parent who knows how to breathe, say 'not today,' and go take a walk around the block just to hear their own thoughts again.

Because when you run on fumes, everything feels like a crisis. The spilled juice becomes a meltdown. The unanswered "Mom?" or "Dad?" feels like a personal attack. The normal chaos of parenting starts sounding like disrespect, and before you know it, you're reacting to your own exhaustion, not their behavior. You don't need more willpower, you need more capacity. And capacity comes from rest, boundaries, and being honest about what you can actually give.

Your children are watching you. Not just how you love them, but how you love yourself. They're learning whether rest is allowed, whether needs can be spoken, whether saying no is a betrayal or a boundary. So take that nap, take that long shower, take back your peace in pieces if you have to. Because your wholeness isn't a luxury, it's actually a legacy.

What I've Seen

Taking trips is something everyone in my family enjoys. My wife and I have always made it a priority to take our kids on therapeutic getaways whenever we could. I also made sure she and I had opportunities to travel without the kids, so we could have some adult time. But I noticed something, as soon as the plane landed or when we checked into our room, she would immediately bring up the kids. At first, it infuriated me. But then I'd take a breath and remind myself that no matter where we were in the world, she would always be "mama bear." Even though I wanted the trip to be kid-free and stress-free, her motherly instincts always seemed to kick in, especially at the gift shops. During excursions, moments of joy would suddenly shift into, "I bet the kids would've loved this, I wonder what they're up to, I'm going to call them."

It took me a while to realize that she wasn't trying to ruin the moment, she was living in both worlds at once. That's what so many mothers do. Even in rest, their minds are multitasking. Even in joy, they're scanning for who's missing. And while I craved disconnection from the day-to-day, she was wired to stay connected. It wasn't about control at all, it was about care. And instead of resenting it, I had to learn how to hold space for both of us, to honor her need to check in and protect our time to check out. Because being a parent doesn't mean you stop being partners. And the health of our relationship deserves just as much intentionality as the way we raise our kids.

That realization didn't just change how I viewed our time as a couple, it also changed how I showed up for myself. Because if I was going to give my kids the best of me, I had to learn how to protect the parts of me that needed refueling. Something that most fathers never truly get to experience without feeling guilty.

One Saturday I had planned a 'solo-dolo' errand run. Nothing fancy. Just me, my music, getting an oil change, and an hour and a half of peace. But when I grabbed my keys, my six year old daughter asked, "Where are you going? I wanted to play Uno." Guilt stabbed me like a steak knife. I almost stayed. But instead, I knelt down and said,

"I love playing Uno with you, in fact it's one of my favorite games. But I also need a break so I can come back with more energy to enjoy it." She nodded. I left. I returned refreshed. We played Uno. And I won of course. Twice!

Another time, I snapped over spilled juice. Not because of the juice, but because I hadn't eaten, showered, or sat down all day. I wasn't tired from parenting, I was tired from abandoning myself in the name of parenting. Obviously it's easier to see these truths in reflection rather than real time. But through reflection is when we pause, listen, and learn. Yes we must take care of our children, but our children love us more when we take care of ourselves.

I'll admit, in the early days of parenthood, anytime I stepped out with my friends, guilt hit me like clockwork. Even if I was just sitting at Applebee's with my fraternity brothers, laughing over wings and watching the game, my mind was somewhere else. I kept wondering what my kids were doing, if they missed me, if they were upset. Did they feel abandoned? I wasn't gone for long, but the weight of being away felt heavy, like I was betraying them by needing time for myself.

On the flip side, when I was home with my kids, I often felt drained mentally, emotionally, and spiritually. I craved a break like it was oxygen. And that inner tug-of-war, that inner see-saw, only added to the confusion. Why is it that when I'm with my kids, I feel overwhelmed and desperate for space, but the moment I get that space, all I can think about is them? Cue the dramatic hair pull. It was like no matter where I was, part of me felt like I was failing at something.

That's the paradox of parenthood no one warns you about, the ability to feel two opposite things at the exact same time. Love and overwhelm. Gratitude and frustration. Devotion and a deep desire to just be alone for five minutes. It's not a sign that you're broken or ungrateful. It simply means that you're human. And part of emotional self-regulation is learning how to hold space for those contradictions without shaming yourself for them.

You don't need to choose between being a present parent and being a person with limits. You can honor both. You can sit in the messy middle, where joy and exhaustion coexist, and still show up with love, grace, and boundaries. The goal isn't to eliminate the tension. The goal is to get comfortable living in it without losing yourself.

That guilt taught me something I didn't know I needed to learn. Somewhere along the line, I had started shrinking myself down to just a one-role parent. And while parenting is sacred, it's not supposed to swallow your entire identity. You are allowed to be a parent and a person. You are allowed to laugh with your friends, pursue your passions, take a night off, go on a trip, or sit in silence doing absolutely nothing, not as an escape, but as an act of wholeness.

The fact is, your children don't need a version of you who's constantly sacrificing, apologizing, or proving your love by disappearing into their needs. They need to see what it looks like to live fully, with purpose and with joy. The more you show up for yourself, the more space you create for them to do the same in their own lives. Reclaiming your identity shouldn't feel like neglect, it should feel like leadership.

Looking back, I realize that guilt wasn't coming from my kids, it was coming from me. From the pressure I put on myself to be everything, all the time. From the belief that good parents don't need breaks. That if I truly loved my kids, I wouldn't want space. But love and space can exist together. In fact, they have to. Because when I deny myself presence, rest, or joy, I'm not actually giving more to my kids, I'm giving them a version of me that's running on fumes and guilt, not grace. And that's not sustainable. For them or for me.

Why We Feel Guilt

As a child, I didn't have many opportunities to go on trips. Not because my parents didn't love me, they simply couldn't afford it. I wanted to see my favorite baseball team, the Atlanta Braves. I wanted to go to Disney World. I dreamed of flying on an airplane. But I wouldn't experience any of those things until I became an adult.

So when I had children of my own, my conscience kicked in hard. I never wanted them to feel the lack of experiences I grew up with. That's why, even now, if I travel without them or find myself enjoying something as simple as a juicy veggie burger, I'm immediately hit with guilt, thinking about what they might be missing out on.

But what I've come to understand is that giving my kids more doesn't mean I have to give them everything, all the time.

Providing new experiences shouldn't come at the cost of my own joy. Honestly, part of breaking generational cycles isn't just giving them what we didn't have, it's also learning to enjoy what we never had, without feeling guilty. Because if I can't allow myself to savor a moment, take a trip, or bite into something delicious without thinking I'm depriving them, then I'm still parenting from a place of remorse. And I don't want to pass that scarcity mindset down, not through my wallet, and not through my emotional habits. They deserve abundance. And dammit, so do I.

I've spent years trying to give my kids the world. The trips, the memories, and the moments I never had. And I don't regret a second of it. But I've also learned that giving doesn't mean disappearing. I've also learned that joy isn't a limited resource. That it's okay for them to see me laugh without them, eat without them, breathe without them, and still know they are deeply, undeniably loved. Because I'm not just raising children, I'm raising myself too. And if abundance is what I want for them, then I have to start living like I deserve it too.

We grew up watching parents sacrifice everything, joy, dreams, and identity, for the family. If you're a mom, the world claps when you disappear for everyone else. If you're a dad showing up emotionally and taking time for yourself, society still acts like it's a miracle or a luxury.

We weren't taught that boundaries are healthy. We were taught that being "good" means being exhausted. An absurd notion. Almost as ridiculous as being told that grinding eighty hours a week and skipping sleep is the secret to success, not a shortcut to a meltdown. There are plenty of times when you've said "yes" even though your body has said "no."

How This Shows Up

- Saying yes when your body is screaming no.
- Snapping at your child because you haven't slept.
- Feeling guilty for resting, eating alone, or saying 'not now'.
- Feeling like your needs are inconvenient.

Try this exercise: Say This, Not That

Say This, 'I matter too. The dishes can wait.'
Not That, 'I'll rest when everything's done.'
Say This, 'Time for me helps me show up better for you.'
Not That, 'I feel bad taking time away.'
Say This, 'I'm making time because I deserve it.'
Not That, 'I don't have time for myself.'

The Mirror Moment

Your child doesn't just need you to be present, they need you whole. Every time you model rest, you're teaching them that rest is something you don't have to earn, that boundaries are beautiful, and that love doesn't mean depletion. You're not abandoning them when you care for yourself. You're protecting them from your burnout.

There were times when I would raise my voice at my children in anger and irritation. Mostly it was because I was tired and worn out. That's when I realized, managing my emotions isn't just self-control, it's protection. Self-care is truly self-love. My cup shouldn't have to go bare because I'm pouring into theirs. Because whenever I show up empty, I find myself parenting from frustration instead of intention. And that's definitely not the legacy I want to leave behind. I want them to remember a parent who paused, who took a breath, who took care of himself so he could take care of them better. Not perfectly, but fully. Consistently. Lovingly. With a heart that wasn't just surviving, but also healing.

You need to know you're not selfish for resting. You're not weak for needing space. You're not a bad parent for saying 'not right now.' You're a person. Still growing. Still healing. Still worthy. And when your child sees you care for yourself, they will grow up knowing that they can do the same.

The day will come when they won't just remember what you gave them, they'll also remember how you treated yourself. They'll remember if you smiled for real, or if it was forced through fatigue. They'll remember if rest was something you respected, or something you resented. And they'll carry that into their own lives, into their own parenting.

So give them the gift of watching you choose peace. Let them see you protect your joy. Show them that love doesn't mean losing yourself, it means returning to yourself, over and over again, with grace. When they see you rest they learn that they don't have to break themselves to be loved. That their needs matter too. They need to know that burnout isn't a glorious triumph. You are modeling a healthy adulthood. Don't just tell them to take care of themselves, show them how.

Reflection + Challenge

1. What's one small thing I feel guilty for doing just for me?
2. Where did that guilt come from?
3. What do I want my child to believe about self-worth and self-care?
4. What's one way I can care for myself this week without apology?

Challenge: Schedule something restorative this week: a nap, a walk, a book, a solo meal, and do it guilt-free. Then talk to your kids about why you did it.

The Amen

I'll say it again, and even louder for the people in the back, you can't pour from an empty vessel. Choosing yourself isn't selfish, it's a must. Rest, refill, and return whole. Your family will thank you for it. Learning to recognize your triggers, and knowing when your mind and body need a break, is a form of wisdom. Take the pause without punishing yourself. Step away before you burn out. Those small moments of intentional rest are far more valuable than reaching a breaking point and becoming unavailable to the people who need you most. You don't have to disappear to be present, you just need to protect your peace to show up fully.

5

Thou Shalt Not Pass Trauma to Thy Own Children

Call It What It Is

You can easily pass down what you haven't healed. You can't protect your children from trauma if you're still parenting through your own. Unhealed trauma doesn't just disappear, it disguises itself, as control, as perfectionism, as yelling, as silence, as fear dressed up as protection. If you don't interrupt the cycle, you will repeat it, even with the best intentions.

My father often seemed angry, and he drowned himself in alcohol. As a child, I saw only an angry, drunken man. But with age came understanding. Maybe he was carrying something much heavier. His drinking was likely a way to cope, to escape a reality shaped by pain. I wanted to believe he had dreams. I wanted to believe he wanted more for himself, and for us. But the trauma his parents carried may have been passed down to him, and in turn, passed down to us.

I now realize that unspoken pain becomes a blueprint. It shapes how we love, how we discipline, how we connect. My father didn't talk about what hurt him, but he lived it. And without knowing it, I started to carry that silence too. Healing, for me, began the moment I stopped asking what was wrong with him, and started asking what happened to him. That moment changed everything.

The cycle doesn't break by accident. It breaks when we choose to do the hard, messy, and necessary work of healing. When we stop running and start feeling, we parent with purpose and not parent from our pain. That's how we reclaim our power. That's how we raise our children to be free from trauma. And that's how we become the ancestors they'll thank, not the ones they'll have to heal from.

What I've Seen

One day, my child flinched when I raised my voice. Not because I hit them, but because the volume carried something older than me and them. It carried my childhood. It carried memories of anxiety, along with the fear of disappointment. It carried echoes of slammed doors, sharp tones, and the kind of tension that makes you hold your breath even when no one's touching you. And they felt it. That moment stopped me in my tracks. My child wasn't reacting to me, they were reacting to the ghosts I hadn't dealt with. And I realized, you don't have to lay hands to pass down harm. Sometimes, all it takes is your tone and your energy.

Another time, I watched my son bottle his feelings. When I asked him why, he said, "I didn't want to make you mad." I hadn't even raised my voice, but my mood had shifted. He could feel it. The unspoken tension, the emotional shutdown, the silence that comes before the storm. That's when I realized, my trauma was living rent-free in my reactions and my kids were paying the cost. Every time I swallowed an emotion instead of processing it, every time I reacted from fear instead of love, I was giving my kids a version of me I hadn't even chosen, it was just the one I inherited.

So now, I choose differently. I choose to feel, to pause, to unlearn. I choose to notice when my volume isn't about the moment, but about the memories. I choose to specifically name what hurt me, so it won't keep hiding in my parenting. This work is not easy at all, but I know it's needed and necessary. Because every time I heal a part of myself, I'm protecting a part of them. I'm raising children who won't have to recover from me. And that is the real cycle break.

Why This Happens

We were raised to survive and not to feel. "Be quiet." "Be tough." "Don't talk about that." So now, when our kids express their feelings or challenge us, it triggers parts of us that were never allowed to exist. We say things like, "You're too sensitive," or "Stop crying, it's not that bad," or "When I was your age, I didn't have time for emotions." But trauma isn't just the hard thing that happened, it's what lingers when the healing didn't. And silence? That's how it spreads.

How This Shows Up

- Yelling over small things.
- Withdrawing when triggered.
- Treating emotions as threats.
- Repeating harmful phrases or discipline styles.
- Overreacting to your child's independence or voice.

Try this exercise: Say This, Not That

Say This, 'I see you're upset. I'm here when you're ready to talk.'

Not That, 'Stop crying or I'll give you something to cry about.'

Say This, 'Tell me what you're feeling.'

Not That, 'You're being dramatic.'

Say This, 'I need a moment, but we'll come back to this.'

Not That, 'I don't want to talk about it.'

The Mirror Moment

Healing doesn't mean you never mess up. It means you recognize the moment, take a beat, and choose differently. Cycle-breaking parenting can be difficult, but it's righteous and rewarding. Every time you breathe instead of scream, explain instead of shame, hug instead of shut down, you are parenting your child and re-parenting yourself. That's generational work.

The cycle doesn't break by accident. It breaks when you decide that survival isn't enough and you want to thrive. It breaks when you give yourself permission to grieve what you never got to and promise to give your children something better. Not perfect, just honest. Not pain-free, just aware. That is the generational shift. You stop bleeding on people who didn't cut you. You stop handing down silence like a family heirloom. And you show your children that real strength is actually healing your pain and not hiding it or running from it.

Reflection + Challenge

1. What phrase or discipline habit am I repeating from childhood?
2. What emotion or behavior triggers me more than it should?
3. What did I need as a child that I didn't get, and how can I

give that to my own child now?
4. What does healing look like in my parenting this week?

Challenge: When you're triggered, pause. Take one breath. Ask, "Am I responding to my child or my own past?" Then simply respond, don't react.

Signs You're Healing the Cycle

- You pause before reacting.
- You apologize when you're wrong.
- You validate their emotions even when they frustrate you.
- You get curious instead of controlling.

For myself, this is what change looks and feels like. It's not loud and over-bearing. It's just simply consistent.

The Amen

Ignoring your past trauma doesn't make it go away. Trust me! It only stores it in a pressure cooker, waiting to explode. Allow yourself the space and freedom to acknowledge it without guilt or shame. Naming what hurt you isn't weakness, it's wisdom. Because once you see it clearly, you can choose not to pass it on. And that choice? That's where healing begins.

You are not your trauma. You are not your past. You are not your parents' pain. You are the interrupter. You are the healer. The new beginning. And your children? They'll get to grow up whole because you chose to do the work, even when you were broken. That is true strength and that is true parenting.

6

Thou Shalt Listen to Thy Children

Call It What It Is

Listening is not waiting for your turn to speak. It's not nodding while planning your rebuttal. It's not interjecting and correcting every sentence mid-breath. Listening is an act of love. And in this world, where kids are surrounded by noise, influence, content, ads, and digital chaos, what they need most is a parent who truly hears them.

I'll admit, when you're the grown-up now, with bills, fatigue, and your own inner noise, it's easy to forget what it feels like to be small and unheard. It's easy to dismiss their complaints or cut them off with "Because I said so." But I remember being that child, the one who just wanted someone to take their feelings seriously, even if they didn't make sense yet. And now that I'm the parent, I realize those tiny voices don't get louder when ignored, they just get quieter. And that silence grows into distance.

So now, I choose to listen with my whole self, not just with my ears, but with my patience, my presence, and my empathy. I remind myself that every "silly" story, every long-winded explanation, and every emotional outburst is a doorway into their world. And when I take the time to truly hear them, I'm not just parenting, I'm building trust. I'm teaching them that their voice matters, and that home is the first place where they'll always be seen, heard, and understood.

What I've Seen

My son once came home from school quiet. I asked him if everything was okay. He said yes, but something felt off. Instead of pushing, I sat next to him and said, "I'm here if you want to talk. No rush." Fifteen minutes later, he opened up. Turns out someone made a joke at his expense, and he didn't know how to process it. He just needed to know I'd listen without flipping out.

That moment marked the beginning of my journey toward listening with greater intention. With five daughters, I knew this was a skill I couldn't afford to overlook. Each of them would have their own stories, some laced with drama, others with sadness or disappointment, and many filled with joy and excitement. They'd want to share those moments with me, not for advice or correction, but for connection. And I needed to be the kind of father who could hold space for them, without judgment, without interruption, and without intimidation.

For the record, when you create a safe place for your children to speak, you become their first example of what being emotionally safe feels like. You're not just listening to stories, you're shaping their self-worth and building their confidence, along with their sense of belonging. And in a world that will try to silence them, second-guess them, and shame them, your home should be the one place where their voices don't just echo, they land.

I knew my efforts had started to bear fruit once both of my daughters reached high school, the same high school where I happened to be a teacher. Despite the potential awkwardness of seeing their dad walking the halls among them and their friends, we had built a relationship rooted in trust and openness. I had created a space where they felt safe coming to me about the realities of their world, the joys, the drama, the fears, even the subjects that made me squirm. Yes, that included parties and boys. But instead of shutting down or reacting in fear, I reminded myself, this is the reward of intentional parenting, access. Not just to their stories, but to their hearts.

The goal was never to control their choices, but to earn their confidence. To be the one they came to first, not last. And even in the moments that tested me most, I held on to that. Because if they can talk to me about the hard stuff now, they'll know they can come to me later, when the stakes are even higher, and the world is even louder. That's the kind of bond I prayed for. That's the kind of father I'm still becoming.

Why It's Hard to Really Listen

We were raised in homes where children were seen, not heard. Where questioning meant disrespect. Where silence was safer than honesty. So now, when our kids talk back, talk too much, or talk about things we weren't allowed to, we shut down or overreact. What I learned from experience, when a child feels unheard at home, they'll go elsewhere to feel seen.

How This Shows Up

- Cutting kids off mid-sentence.
- Listening to fix, not to understand.

- Invalidating their feelings ("You're fine.")
- Dismissing their experiences as "just kid stuff."
- Reacting with lectures instead of curiosity.

Try this exercise: Say This, Not That

Say This, "It may seem small to me, but it's clearly big to you. Let's talk about it."

Not That, "That's not a big deal."

Say This, "You're feeling this deeply, let's figure out what's underneath it."

Not That, "You're being dramatic."

Say This, "I want to help you understand now, let's walk through it together."

Not That, 'You'll understand when you're older."

The Mirror Moment

When your child speaks and you listen, I mean really listen, you're doing more than gathering information. You are teaching them that their voice matters, that emotions are not emergencies, that their thoughts are safe in your presence. You're not just hearing them, you are shaping their self-worth.

The goal is for this behavior to transfer when they're not with me. Prayerfully, our children will learn how to listen and communicate even when they're angry, without shutting down or lashing out, and without letting charged emotions lead the way. I want them to know that feeling something deeply isn't a weakness, and neither is taking a pause to process before responding. That kind of emotional regulation is a gift, and it's one they'll carry far beyond our home.

Because one day, they'll be out in the world, in classrooms, boardrooms, relationships, and eventually parenting rooms of their own. And when conflict arises, I hope they'll hear my voice in their head saying, "Slow down. Breathe. Listen to understand, not to win." Not because I was perfect, but because I practiced what I wanted them to learn. Because I didn't just preach peace, I actually modeled it.

That's the legacy of listening. It doesn't stop at home. It follows them into adulthood. It becomes a part of who they are and how they love. And if that's the only thing they carry forward from me, a soft heart, steady ears, and the courage to stay present in hard moments, I'll know I did something right.

What They're Really Saying (When You Listen Closely)

- "I don't want to go to school" might mean "I'm overwhelmed."
- "Nobody likes me" might mean "I feel invisible."
- "Leave me alone" might mean "I don't know how to ask for connection."

Listening is more than hearing the words they speak, it's decoding the heart behind them.

Reflection + Challenge

1. Do I tend to fix, teach, or interrupt before fully hearing my child?
2. What does 'active listening' look like in my parenting?
3. When was the last time I really listened without reacting?
4. What's one small habit I can change this week to listen better?

Challenge: Next time your child shares something, pause. Reflect back on what you heard before responding. Watch how they light up when they feel understood.

The Amen

Your child doesn't need a perfect parent, they need a safe one. They need a place where their voice doesn't have to compete with your stress, your ego, or your assumptions. Let your ears be soft, open not just to their words but to the feelings behind them. Let your words be few, because sometimes silence speaks louder than advice. Let your presence be strong, not intimidating, but anchoring. A calm in their chaos. A steady in their storm. Because when your child feels truly heard in the small things, they'll come to you with the big things. And when you listen to them now, with patience, without panic, they'll be more likely to listen to your wisdom later. Not because they had to, but because they wanted to. Because they trusted you.

7

Thou Shalt Not Let Technology Raise Thy Own

Call It What It Is

As usual let's keep it all the way real, screens are raising a lot of children right now. And truthfully, that's not brand new. Even back in the '90s, the television was my babysitter and part-time guardian more times than I can count. The Brady Bunch, The Cosby Show, and In Living Color were shows that felt like extended family members. But today, it's gone next-level. YouTube is the babysitter. TikTok is the reckless older cousin handing out bad advice. Netflix is the bedtime storyteller. And Google? That's the grand-parent or older relative in the house with all the answers.

It's not because we don't care, it's because we're exhausted. Outnumbered. Distracted. Overwhelmed. Sometimes we just need a moment of peace, and handing them a screen buys us that moment.

But here's the warning label, whatever grabs their attention starts shaping their values. Every scroll, every video, every viral "joke," it's planting seeds. About beauty. About relationships.

About identity. About what's normal. And if we're not guiding those conversations, the internet will. Not with wisdom. Not with love. But with algorithms. And algorithms don't care about character, they only care about clicks.

What I've Seen

One day, I heard my eight-year-old daughter say she felt sad and depressed. When her mother and I gently asked why, what was wrong, she couldn't give us an answer. At first, we were confused. But after digging a little deeper, we discovered she had recently started watching shows designed for pre-teens. These shows centered around big emotions like sadness, anxiety, and depression. In that particular moment, I wasn't sure if she was truly feeling those things from within, if she had connected with something familiar, or if she was being led to feel that way by what she was absorbing.

It raised a deeper question. How much of our children's emotional world is theirs, and how much is borrowed from the media they consume?

One afternoon, I was grabbing a quick nap while the baby slept and the girls were playing. Their mom was at work, and I'd been holding it down solo all day. Suddenly, the house filled with blaring sound, the TV volume turned all the way up. I jumped up, disoriented and frustrated, only to find my daughters laughing and pretending the remote didn't work. It was a prank, something they'd seen on YouTube and decided to recreate.

I was furious. Not just because my nap was interrupted or because I was scared the baby would wake up, but because I realized something deeper, my kids were being taught what's funny, what's normal, and what's acceptable by the internet.

That moment hit me hard. These weren't just silly jokes anymore. The digital world was shaping their worldview, and if I didn't stay present and intentional, I'd be letting algorithms raise them. And as a content creator myself, I couldn't ignore my own role in the system. We're not just parenting in the digital age, we're competing with it, feeding it, and trying to protect our kids from it, all at the same time.

Another time, I brought one of my daughters to an important meeting. To keep her quiet and occupied, I handed her an iPad without thinking twice. It worked, she stayed distracted. But afterward, I felt uneasy. What was I teaching her? That silence must be filled with screens? That it's not normal to sit still and wait? In trying to manage the moment, I may have missed the lesson.

And it reminded me again, sometimes, parenting isn't about convenience. It's about consciousness.

That's why we can't afford to check out. We don't have to be perfect, tech-free parents living off the grid, but we do have to be present. We have to be the ones who put context around the content. The ones who ask, "What did you think about that video?" or "How did that make you feel?" We have to pause and say, "That's not how we treat people," or "That's not true, here's what is."

We have to become interpreters along with being enforcers. Because the goal isn't to shelter them from the world, it's to equip them to live in it without losing themselves. And that means being there, staying curious, and choosing connection over convenience, even when we're tired.

Why It Happens

We use tech because it's like fast food, convenient. It's also quiet and familiar. And when we're busy or burned out, screens become survival. But let's not pretend the algorithm is neutral. These apps are built to hook. To numb. To teach our kids without asking permission. If you don't raise your child, the algorithm will. And there have been numerous cases where the outcome hasn't always been positive.

How This Shows Up

- Screens during every meal.
- Meltdowns when it's time to turn it off.
- Quoting influencers more than parents.
- Obsession with likes, followers, and trends.
- Losing interest in offline life.

Say This, Not That

Say This, "Here's 30 minutes to chill. Then we're going outside together."

Not That, "Fine, just watch something so I can work."

Say This, "I miss you. Let's do something without screens for a bit."

Not That, "Why are you always on that phone?"

Say This, "Let's learn how to use it without letting it use us."

Not That, "Technology is ruining kids."

The Mirror Moment

Technology is not the enemy. But it is a tool, and tools can either build or break. We don't have to ban everything. We just have to be present enough to guide it and filter it.

Your attention is more powerful than any app. Your presence can outshine any screen. And your love can't be downloaded, it must be lived.

If you haven't been as present as you'd like, or if it feels like the car's already too far down the driveway, let me remind you, it's never too late to jump back in. What happened before doesn't define you. What you choose to do from this moment forward does.

If you're unfamiliar with social media, learn it with your child. Ask questions. Get curious. See what they're watching, what they love, what's shaping their humor, their interests, their identity. This isn't about control at all, it's about connection.

It's a chance to step into their world, side by side, instead of from behind a wall of rules, fear, or tradition.

Because when your child sees that you care enough to meet them where they are, not to judge, but to understand, you build trust. And trust is what gives your voice power in a noisy world.

You don't need to know every trend or app to make an impact. You just need to show up, listen without overreaction, and remind them through your presence, they're not alone in this.

Reflection + Challenge

1. When do I default to screens instead of connection?
2. What's one area where technology has taken too much space in our home?
3. How can I model a healthy relationship with my own devices?
4. What's one offline moment I can create this week?

Challenge: Designate one tech-free time block this week, meals, car rides, or bedtime. Let your child lead the conversation. See what comes up when the scrolling stops.

Remember: They don't need constant entertainment. They need to feel like they matter more than the device in your hand.

The Amen

One day, they'll outgrow cartoons and tablets and trends. But they'll remember who sat down next to them. Who asked questions. Who turned the phone off and leaned in. Let tech supplement, not substitute. Let your love be louder than the noise. And show them, human connection will always be the main character.

8

Thou Shalt Not Gossip Around Thy Children

Call It What It Is

Kids don't just overhear us. They absorb us. They soak up our tone, sarcasm, body language, side-eyes, and shade, even when we think they're not paying attention. What you say about other people becomes part of how your child understands love, loyalty, trust, and conflict. Gossiping around your kids could become dangerous, and they can grow up thinking disrespect is a love language.

Let's keep it a buck as always, not every conversation is meant for children's ears. Especially the ones loaded with adult themes, heavy emotions, or inappropriate content. Some topics are simply too complex or explicit for their stage of understanding. When we speak carelessly around our kids, we risk introducing them to concepts they're not emotionally equipped to process. It plants confusion. Suddenly, they're holding pieces of a conversation they don't fully understand, and in that confusion, their minds start to fill in the gaps. What begins as curiosity quickly turns into worry, misunderstanding, or even fear.

That's why mindful communication is a form of protection. Our kids are always listening, even when we think they're not. We owe it to them to create emotional boundaries with our words, just like we would with our actions. In no way am I saying hide the world from them, instead I'm saying we should guide them through it in ways their hearts and minds can handle. When we speak with intention, we don't protect their innocence only, we also preserve their trust.

What I've Seen

"Children don't sit around grown folks when they're talking." That phrase echoed throughout my childhood, passed down like a commandment at every family gathering. The adults would post up in the living room, laughing loud, dancing, swapping stories, sipping something strong, while all the kids were either squeezed into a back bedroom or sent outside to play, weather permitting. We'd press our ears to the walls or walk past the door hoping to catch a glimpse of what felt like a secret club. But honestly? It was kind of nice staying in kid territory, doing back flips in the grass, playing tag, or minding children's business with other children who didn't care about bills or breakups.

Still, there were other times, quiet, tense moments, when my parents would talk behind closed doors, thinking I couldn't hear them. But I did. I'd catch fragments, emotions, whispered arguments, and I'd fill in the blanks with my imagination. Slowly, piece by piece, I built my own version of the story, whether it was accurate or not. That's the thing about children, even when we're not talking to them, we're still talking around them. And they absorb it all, the tone, the tension, the truth between the lines. That's why being intentional with our conversations isn't just about what they hear, it's about what they carry.

Honestly, most of the inappropriate things I learned growing up didn't come from TV or the internet, they came from school. When I got around my friends, they'd casually repeat things they overheard their parents say. And let me tell you, some of it made my jaw drop. I knew I wasn't supposed to be hearing it, but I couldn't stop listening. It was wild, messy, and completely unfiltered. If my parents had known the kind of conversations floating around the fourth-grade lunch table and playground, they would've had a fit.

As parents, we have to keep this in mind. When we speak openly, and carelessly, around children, we have no control over where that information will land next. Their little ears soak it in, and their little mouths repeat it in places we'd never expect. When I became a teacher, I saw it firsthand. I knew who was sleeping with who, who had just gotten out of jail, and who owed someone money, all from the mouths of elementary and middle school children. It made me hyper-aware of what I say around my own children. Because I started wondering, how much of what they're repeating is misunderstood? How much of it is half-true? And how much of it is just plain damaging?

That's why it matters. What we say doesn't just stay in the room, it travels. Through hallways, classrooms, and playground whispers. And before you know it, a private adult conversation has become public playground gossip. Our children don't just carry our words, they spread them. So let's be mindful of the seeds we plant, because once they take root, we can't always control where they grow.

Why It Happens

Some of us grew up in homes where gossip was the family

sport. Where tea was currency. Where throwing shade was a bonding ritual. We weren't taught to process. We were taught to whisper, to judge, and to perform politeness while holding onto resentment. When we do that around our kids, we teach them that love is conditional and trust is performative.

How This Shows Up

- Talking about family members or neighbors in a critical way.
- Sarcastic or passive-aggressive comments kids repeat later.
- Using your child as a sounding board or emotional dumping ground.
- Teaching double standards, "be kind" but modeling the opposite.

Try this exercise: Say This, Not That

Say This, She brings a lot of energy into the room.'

Not That, 'She's always doing the most.'

Say This, 'He's figuring things out. Let's keep an eye out without judging.'

Not That, 'That boy is bad news.'

Say This, 'I'm feeling unappreciated, I think we need to talk it out.'

Not That, 'After everything I've done for them...'

The Mirror Moment

You don't have to pretend everything is perfect. But you do have to ask: Would I be okay if my child repeated this in public? When we model honest communication without pettiness, we give our kids the emotional tools to build strong relationships, not messy circles and cycles.

Reflection + Challenge

1. What types of conversations do I have when my children are nearby?
2. Have they ever repeated something I said that made me cringe?
3. Am I using sarcasm, gossip, or shame as humor?
4. What would change if I made kindness the default tone in my home?

Challenge: Go one week without talking negatively about anyone around your child. If you slip, name it and repair it, out loud. If there's a conversation that needs to be had, send them away or remove yourself from the room.

What They Learn When You Gossip

- "Love is earned and lost quickly."
- "People talk behind your back."
- "Being critical = being close."

Flip the script and show them:

- Love stays kind, even when disappointed.
- You can vent without disrespect.
- Home is a safe space, not a petty stage.

The Amen

You don't have to be perfect with your words. But you do have to be intentional. Let your child grow up knowing you don't joke at other people's expense. That they shouldn't find humor in humiliation. You protect people's dignity even when they're not present. You choose peace over performance. Because what they hear now becomes how they speak later. That's real talk.

9

Thou Shalt Take Accountability and Apologize When in Wrong

Call It What It Is

A lot of us were raised by people who never said, "I apologize" nor "I'm sorry," not because they didn't love us, but because they didn't see apology as a tool. They saw it as a weakness. But accountability is not a weakness, it is actually strength wrapped in vulnerability. And when you can say "I was wrong" to your child, you're not losing authority, you're gaining trust. Apologies teach emotional safety, and safety builds strong children.

What I've Seen

Have you ever yelled at, or punished, your child for something, only to find out later they didn't actually do it? That awkward, gut-sinking feeling? Yeah, I've been there more than once. Early in my parenting journey, I'd sometimes just keep it moving, too proud or unsure of how to handle the mistake. But as my children got older, and as I grew wiser, I learned something important, it's okay to admit when you're wrong. In fact, it's necessary. I started making it a point to apologize when I messed up, because I realized that accountability isn't just something I teach my children, it's something I have to model.

A few years ago, I dropped my teenagers off at the skating rink for teen night. Unfortunately, a fight broke out, and several children got involved. My daughter sent me a few videos of the chaos, and I was instantly furious. Not because of the fight itself, but because the footage she sent looked like it had been recorded way too close. I had drilled it into them time and time again: if something breaks out, don't stick around, get out, move away from the crowd. So why did this video look like she had front-row seats?

I called her immediately, angry and anxious, already jumping in the car to pick them up. As soon as they got in, I let loose. No interruptions, just a full-on parental soliloquy about how they knew better. And when I finally stopped, my daughter quietly said, "Father, I wasn't near the fight. Someone sent that to me." Whew! If I could've melted into the driver's seat, I would've. I was embarrassed, but also relieved. Relieved that they had actually listened, that they were safe. But I could see it on their faces, the hurt, the disappointment that I hadn't even asked first. I apologized right away. Because in that moment, I was reminded again that parenting is about learning, too. Sometimes we get it wrong, and when we do, we have to make it right.

That moment stayed with me, not because I messed up, but because I chose to own it. Our kids don't need us to be flawless. They need to see what humility looks like. They need to know that love isn't just loud when they're wrong, but it's just as loud when we are too. Every time we apologize, we're not losing authority, we're gaining trust. And that trust becomes the bridge they'll walk across when life gets harder, and the stakes get higher. Accountability doesn't weaken our role as parents, it strengthens the bond that holds the whole relationship together.

Why It's Hard

We weren't taught how to apologize. We were taught how to assert dominance, save face, and move on. We heard you're too sensitive, it wasn't that serious, and get over it you'll be fine. But the absence of accountability creates a presence of resentment, and silence becomes another kind of wound.

How This Shows Up

- Yelling without repair.
- Blaming your child for your own reaction.
- Avoiding eye contact or affection after conflict.
- Expecting your child to "move on" while you haven't modeled how.

Try this exercise: Say This, Not That

Say This, "I lost my temper. That's on me."
Not That, "You made me mad."
Say This, "I'm sorry for what I said. It was wrong."
Not That, "I'm sorry you feel that way."
Say This, "I overreacted. Let's try again together."
Not That, "Well, you shouldn't have..."

The Mirror Moment

Your child is not your peer, but they are a person. And when you show them how to own your mistakes, they learn that love is safe even when imperfect. That repair matters more than being right, that it's okay to be wrong and brave enough to make it right. Apologizing doesn't lower your authority, it deepens and strengthens your credibility. And in their world filled with social media, peer pressure, and constant noise, your credibility is more valuable than ever. It's what makes your voice stand out. It's what makes your love believable.

Reflection + Challenge

1. When's the last time I apologized to my child?
2. What made it hard?
3. What messages did I receive about apologizing growing up?
4. What would it look like to model repair more intentionally?

Challenge: The next time you raise your voice, dismiss a feeling, or react from stress, pause. Then return and say, "I was wrong." Watch how powerful those three words are.

When They See You Apologize

- They learn that relationships are repairable.
- They gain language for their own accountability.
- They see that power can be gentle.
- They feel safe, not scared.

You're teaching them how to be whole, and not just obedient.

The Amen

Say it messy, say it late, say it while still figuring it out, just say it. Because one "I'm sorry" today could heal what silence tomorrow would deepen. Model the repair. Be the bridge. Teach the healing. Your legacy will thank you. And when your child grows up and makes their own mistakes, they'll remember what grace looked like. They'll know how to come back, because you showed them how.

10

Thou Shalt Discipline Thy Children and Administer Consequences

Call It What It Is

Let's get this straight, discipline is not a dirty word. It's also not a synonym for punishment, it's not about fear, and it's not about control. Discipline should be about teaching, training, and guidance. When we confuse discipline with punishment, we create fear-based obedience instead of rooted respect. Although fear might get results, it doesn't build relationship. I'm acquainted with this through experience.

So what's the difference between effective discipline and excessive discipline? Shaving a child's head bald because they misbehaved in school and posting it on social media isn't a lesson, it's humiliation. That's not correction, it's public shaming. And while it might grab attention and social engagement, what it really teaches is resentment, embarrassment, and mistrust. That's excessive discipline.

Effective discipline, on the other hand, looks like acknowledging what your child did wrong, having a real conversation about it, and choosing consequences that correct behavior while still preserving their dignity. It's not about making a child pay, it's about helping them grow.

Take this example, a dad comes home and finds his teenage daughter alone in her room with a teenage boy. He loses control, grabs his belt, and aggressively disciplines her, then, to make matters worse, uploads the video to social media. What might have been a teachable moment instead becomes a moment of public shame. Rather than instilling wisdom, he inflicts a wound, not just physical, but emotional. One that says, "You're not safe with me."

Discipline should never come at the cost of trust. It should be rooted in guidance and not control. Love and not fear. But when we use humiliation as artillery in the parenting toolkit, we don't raise stronger children, we raise quieter ones. More disconnected. More cautious with their truth. And that's the opposite of what they really need.

What I've Seen

Anyone who knows me and my dad, knows he didn't play. He wasn't afraid to dish out discipline at any moment, it didn't matter where we were or who was watching. As a kid, I hated it. I couldn't stand the embarrassment or the fear. But as an adult, I began to understand the method behind his madness. His discipline kept me out of major trouble, no doubt. The fear of disappointing him, or worse, the consequences, shaped a lot of my choices. But while his approach kept me in line, it didn't build a deep bond between us. Our relationship wasn't as strong as I wanted it to be.

That's the part I carry with me now as a father. I want my children to respect me, but not out of fear. I want them to feel safe enough to come to me with the hard stuff, and not just obedient when they think I'm watching. Discipline matters, yes, but not at the expense of connection. My goal isn't just to raise well-behaved children, it's to raise emotionally healthy, self-aware humans. Children who know they're loved, even when they mess up. Children who can trust that correction comes from care, not from anger and not from control.

Once I became a father and it was my turn to discipline, I thought I could simply use threats or intimidation to keep my kids in line. But I quickly learned it doesn't work that way. I had to be more intentional. I learned to watch my words, because if I said I was going to do something, I had to follow through. My consistency wasn't just about control, it was about trust, accountability, and credibility. Keeping my word, even in discipline, showed them I meant what I said and that my boundaries weren't just empty warnings.

When it comes to discipline, parents have to hold the line. It's easy to start feeling guilty, like you're being too harsh or letting your child down. I've felt it too. You don't want to be the villain. You want to be their safe space, the one they run to, not the one they fear. But when we blur the line between love and leniency, we unintentionally teach our children that boundaries are optional. If you say no TV for three days, don't cave on day two because they look sad or say all the right things. Discipline without consistency isn't discipline at all, it's a suggestion. And suggestions won't raise children who understand structure, self-control, or consequences.

What we have to remember is that accountability is love. It may not feel good in the moment, for us or for them, but it builds something far more lasting than temporary comfort. Kids don't just need kindness, they need clarity. They need to know that your word means something. That when you say "no," it holds weight. Because one day, the world won't be as forgiving. And your consistency now prepares them to navigate life later. So don't be afraid to be firm. You're not being mean, you're being intentional. And that intention, paired with love, creates real security.

Why It Gets Confusing

Some of us were raised with yelling, threats, and whoopings. While some of us were raised with silence, shame, or manipulation. Very few of us were raised with emotional coaching, logical consequences, or boundaries rooted in connection. So when it's our turn, we either repeat what we know or we freeze because we don't.

How This Shows Up

- Consequences that don't match the behavior.
- Taking everything away out of frustration.
- Confusing control for authority.
- Letting guilt stop you from following through.
- Saying "you're grounded forever!" with no real intention to stick to it.

Try this exercise: Say This, Not That

Say This, "That choice wasn't okay. Let's talk about what happened."

Not That, "You're so bad!"

Say This, "Because you broke the rule, no screen time tonight. We'll try again tomorrow."

Not That, "You're grounded for a month!"

Say This, "I'm frustrated, but I still love you. Let's take a break and come back to this."

Not That, "I'm done with you."

The Mirror Moment

Consequences should teach, not terrify. They should make sense, not just make noise. They should invite reflection, not trigger shame. Your child should walk away from discipline feeling loved, and not broken. Seen, and not scared. And if you mess it up? Circle back. Repair. And try again. That's discipline too.

Sometimes, the most powerful part of discipline isn't the consequence, it's the conversation. It's the quiet moment afterward, when you sit down and reflect with your child. It's when you say, "I'm proud of how you handled that," or "I know that was hard, but I'm glad we talked it through." Discipline isn't always just about correcting the wrong, it's also about building something right. Trust. Communication. Confidence. And that only happens when love stays louder than frustration, and connection becomes the goal, not control.

Reflection + Challenge

1. Do I discipline from calm, or from frustration?
2. Are my consequences logical, consistent, and fair?
3. What's one moment this week where I can guide instead of punish?
4. How can I model the self-control I want to see in my child?

Challenge: Next time your child breaks a rule, pause. Ask yourself: What do I want them to learn from this? Then respond accordingly, with love and with limits.

What Real Discipline Teaches

- Boundaries can be firm and kind.
- Mistakes are part of learning.
- Respect is built, not demanded.
- Love doesn't disappear in hard moments.

This is the type of authority that creates emotionally healthy adults.

The Amen (What We Owe Our Children)

You are not raising robots. You are raising humans. Humans with feelings, questions, and flaws, just like you. Discipline is not about control, it's about coaching in tough moments. It's about preparing your child for a world that won't always be gentle, while showing them that love can be. So teach with clarity. Guide with grace. And when they stumble, stand close. Because when your discipline is rooted in relationship, your child grows up rooted in resilience.

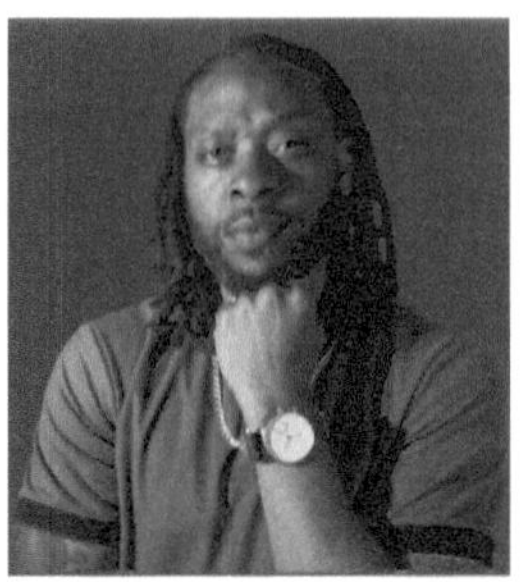

About the Author

About the Author

Leonard McCrary is a father, husband, teacher, music artist, author, and truth-teller. He's not writing this book from a high horse, he's writing it from the kitchen table, between parenting wins and parenting regrets, between a school day and a deep breath.

Raised in a world that didn't always have room for emotional honesty, Leonard chose to break the mold. His life's work is about disrupting cycles, in classrooms, in homes, and in hearts. Whether he's speaking to students, mentoring young men, or creating art that uplifts his community, his message stays the same: healing is possible, and love is the legacy worth fighting for.

Leonard blends humor, wisdom, and real-life storytelling to remind parents that perfection isn't the goal, presence is. Through *The Parent Commandments*, he invites readers to raise children who are not just well-behaved, but well-loved. And to raise themselves in the process.

He currently lives in Chattanooga, TN with his wife and six beautiful children, who continue to teach him more about patience, growth, and unconditional love every single day.

Also by Leonard McCrary

The Parent Commandments is a modern, scripture-style parenting guide written by Leonard McCrary. Blending inspiration, humor, and hard earned wisdom, the book delivers ten powerful lessons designed to help parents heal from their own childhood wounds, build stronger family connections, and break generational cycles. Each "commandment" offers practical reflection, emotional depth, and a call to accountability, empowering readers to lead their homes with love, discipline, and legacy in mind.

www.ingramcontent.com/pod-product-compliance
Lightning Source LLC
LaVergne TN
LVHW090617110826
845146LV00001B/428